the language of healing

daily comfort for women living with breast cancer

the language of healing

daily comfort for women living with breast cancer

pat benson & linda dackman

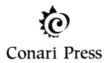

Conari Press

First published in 2014 by Conari Press, an imprint of
Red Wheel/Weiser, LLC
With offices at:
665 Third Street, Suite 400
San Francisco, CA 94107
www.redwheelweiser.com

ISBN: 978-1-57324-631-6

Library of Congress Cataloging-in-Publication Data
Benson, Pat.
  The language of healing : daily comfort for women living with breast
cancer / Pat Benson and Linda Dackman.
     pages cm
  ISBN 978-1-57324-631-6
 1. Breast--Cancer. 2. Breast--Cancer--Patients. I. Dackman, Linda.
II. Title.
  RC280.B8B44 2014
  616.99'449--dc23

                    2013048181

Cover design by Jim Warner
Cover photograph © shutterstock / daniana
Interior by Jane Hagaman
Typeset in Constantia

Printed on acid-free paper in the United States of America.
EBM
10 9 8 7 6 5 4 3 2 1
The paper used in this publication meets the minimum requirements
of the American National Standard for Information Sciences—Perma-
nence of Paper for Printed Library Materials Z39.48-1992 (R1997).

Some people see scars, and it is the wounding they remember. To me, they are proof that there is healing.

Linda K. Hogan

Contents

Foreword

"Breast cancer," the doctor said to my frightened mother as I looked on. She wasn't surprised, really. She had felt the lump every day, again and again. Repeatedly, she had run her fingers over it. For many weeks she felt it, she saw it, but she tried to ignore the obvious. And she ignored the voice within too, the voice that said, "Call the doctor." She had not wanted to face the possibility of cancer. She had not wanted her life to change, to know what was on the other side of the lump. Like most women, she simply wanted to wake up one morning and discover the lump gone.

My mother wasn't the only one in the family with breast cancer. My maternal grandmother and three maternal aunts were also diagnosed; five women who faced breast cancer, each in her own way, making different choices, but all bravely meeting the challenges. Every year when I go for my mammogram, I wait, tentatively, for the letter I hope to receive, the one that says, "Your results are normal." I have been lucky, so far. But while we know much more about the genetic links to breast cancer, we also know that the majority of women who get this disease have no family history. A staggering one in eight women will experience breast cancer in her lifetime. And while the medical community has developed more targeted and effective therapies, there is still no cure.

Breast cancer is profoundly painful, most times physically, oftentimes emotionally, and sometimes spiritually. Women come face-to-face with their own mortality, knowing there are no certain outcomes. They turn to other women who are fighting this disease for the support, advice, and inspiration they need. And that is exactly what *The Language of Healing: Daily Comfort for Women Living with Breast Cancer* offers—comfort, guidance, and practical information, from women who have been there.

Pat Benson and Linda Dackman, the authors of this special book of tough and tender reflections, know firsthand the shock of a diagnosis, the grueling challenges of treatment, and the healing power of turning to other women with breast cancer for insight and inspiration. They wanted to offer "a support group in a book," so that help could always be at hand, wherever you are on your journey. *The Language of Healing* includes their voices, as well as the voices of a diverse group of other women of all ages and attitudes. The book is divided into three parts—A Time to Cry, A Time to Heal, and A Time to Live—the portals every woman with breast cancer walks through as she comes to terms with her disease.

I deeply believe that peer support and books are vital tools for healing, so when I was asked to write the foreword to *The Language of Healing*, I was honored. I am the author of a number of books for women who are struggling with a range of life issues. But all my work is grounded in the belief that the path of recovery begins with learning to take life one day at a time, even one moment at a time. This is how we give ourselves the opportunity to listen not only to the "experts," but to consider what our inner voices have to say. This trusting in ourselves, coupled with the open and non-judgmental sharing with other companions on this journey, companions who promise steady, quiet strength, and who can reach us when another's words may ring hollow, who can ease our ways and even change our lives.

The Language of Healing is a companion for you, too, as you walk your individual path on the common ground of breast cancer to arrive at peace. And isn't that what we all want? Regardless of our circumstances, we want the peace to go on moment by moment, and despite whatever has derailed us, the ability to live life fully each day. That resilient spirit of moving through fear, loss, and grief to arrive at such a peace is present on every page of this lovely book.

Karen Casey, author of bestselling books
Each Day a New Beginning and
Change Your Mind and Your Life Will Follow

Thank you to family, friends, and colleagues who supported this project, especially Linda Dackman, Karen Casey, Karen Chernyaev, Jan Johnson, Caroline Pincus, Ken Merz, Jessica Merz Godes, Bryn Benson, and Julie Edstrom. A most special thanks to my grandson, Andrew, for keeping me in the moment, and to the late, great Nick, the best dog ever, for keeping me wild.

Pat Benson

For this book, I wish to acknowledge Pat Benson . . . and Pat Benson only. Thank you, Pat.

Linda Dackman

Introduction

Like so many other women, we, the authors, have lived through the shock of breast cancer diagnoses. One of us was thirty-four years old, a single woman living on the West Coast who had her whole life ahead of her; the other, a post-menopausal, married, fifty-six-year-old Midwesterner, eagerly anticipating the birth of a grandchild. We didn't know each other as we made our separate ways from diagnosis through treatment and recovery. We met when we were asked to explore the possibility of working on a book about confronting breast cancer. We agreed, and as we shared our individual stories, we discovered that while our lives are very different, our breast cancer stories have much in common.

We experienced the same sense of loss and disorientation. We shared similar questions as we wandered through the wilderness of medical opinions, options, choices, and terror. In recovery, we both struggled in the aftermath of the physical, emotional, and psychological effects to our lives. We had to redefine what "normal" meant to us. We began to live life with a renewed sense of the value of each and every day. Most importantly, we found immeasurable support and guidance in listening to the stories of other women facing breast cancer and in sharing ours. By reflecting on the advice and insights offered, we responded to our individual challenges in confident, thoughtful, and healing ways. Acceptance overcame anger, understanding overtook confusion, and courage diminished fear. Moment by moment, breast cancer became an unexpected journey of self-discovery, new friends, and new beginnings.

As we talked more about a potential book, we knew it had to include a diversity of voices, our own as well as those of other women who have a point of view and a deeply felt commitment to helping you on your journey. The result is our personal experiences mingled with those of other women in a down-to-earth volume that is the sum total of many perspectives, interwoven and laid out one upon the other. The scope ranges from the first shock of diagnosis to the ultimately transformative powers of the breast cancer experience—and many of the fears, insights, and even joys in between. You might say that *The Language of Healing* is like a breast cancer support group between the covers of a book. It is exactly what a woman recuperating in her hospital bed or at any of the other milestones of treatment and recovery might need—the accumulated coping devices, insights, wisdom, and inspiration of other women who have preceded her in confronting breast cancer.

Gathered here are moving anecdotes and practical information of value to every woman concerned or diagnosed with this disease. It is built upon the experiences of women of all ages, from twenty-three to eighty-four; women who have undergone all types of breast surgery and treatments, from lumpectomy and mastectomy to radiation and chemotherapy; women who are single, married, divorced, widowed, straight, and gay. The reflections correspond to the progress of varied experiences. Each one begins with a quotation to bring the topic into focus and ends with an affirmation that you may use as guided support in your recovery. You will touch on topics as universal as fear and grief, and as intimate as sexual relations. And you will find wisdom and healing strategies as varied as the individuals who offer them.

Approach this book as you like. Read through it in sequence, or read at random, based on your own shifting questions and needs. However you use it, our hope is that you find *The Language of Healing* to be encouraging and uplifting. It is a place to gain insights into your own experience and discover ways in which others have coped. It is a private place for you to feel supported and understood, a place to share your grief, anger, and sense of loss. Above all, it is a resource to strengthen you in *your* journey of self-discovery as you live moment to moment, with a newly deepened appreciation of life.

Pat Benson and Linda Dackman

Part I.

After Diagnosis
A Time to Cry

Finding Out

Suffering . . . no matter how multiplied . . .
is always individual.

Anne Morrow Lindbergh

What follows a breast cancer diagnosis?

Shock. Disbelief. Fear. Numbness.

The question: "Cancer?"

The answer: "Yes. Cancer."

And then what?

Then you cry.

I let the tears come, the first thing I do for myself.

Shock

Oh Lord! If you but knew
what a brimstone of a creature
I am behind all this beautiful amiability!
Jane Welsh Carlyle

No matter how calm we may appear on the surface, we are standing on unstable ground. No one can absorb the news of breast cancer simply by hearing the diagnosis. The overwhelming reality of it becomes instantly buried under a protective shell of shock.

But reality cracks through our shock, our fear, our denial, little by little, until we are ready to face it. Remember, no matter how together and in control we appear, even to ourselves, we want to respect and acknowledge the chaos beneath.

I acknowledge the chaos underneath the surface
as I struggle to face my diagnosis.

Grief

I tell you hopeless grief is passionless.
Elizabeth Barrett Browning

I have breast cancer, you say to yourself over and over again. Yet you do not fully grasp the meaning of these words. The impact approaches and then recedes, is painfully clear, then muffled. You are inside and outside yourself all at once, aware that something awful has happened, but at the same time you expect to wake up from this terrible dream. You are rocked by shock and fear and grief. Suddenly, you shift. You are above it all, floating calmly, looking down at the world. You see the shattered pieces of yourself on the floor.

I will feel the grief, then gather my energy for moving forward.

Disorientation

Though the body moves, the soul may stay behind.
Murasaki Shikibu

The world moves, our body moves, and our mind rushes off without us, to visit some distant, narrow place at the end of a long, dark tunnel, although our thoughts cannot stay there long.

Our soul stands still, holding on to the world we once knew, the world before we took the word "cancer" inside us, the world we understood before everything changed.

♡

Despite my disorientation, I continue.

Denial

Of course it will never be quite the same.
But what ever is in this life?

Alison Lurie

Cancer sneaks up sideways, quietly. It whispers, sends subtle signals, until it nudges past denial to get our attention. We see the doctors and have the tests. Whether the results are delivered gently or roughly, the diagnosis is clear— breast cancer.

The bad news settles on the surface. We can't fathom our death, and we can't fathom living with this disease. We sit quietly, unable to find the words to comfort ourselves, or the people we love. There are next steps to be taken. But we're not ready to be brave, or to let go of our old life, and accept this news.

I give myself time to accept this diagnosis and the changes it will bring.

Anger

*I'm so angry that my body is
all but bursting into flame.*

Alamanda

The anger we feel is terrifying, directed as it is against the very universe. The anger within is sudden, wrenching. We scream, "How dare this happen to me?"

We are raging against the implication that our lives as we have known them are about to be destroyed. We are burning with anger at the threat to our plans, our expectations, to our very future.

Think of this anger as an erupting volcano, because from the volcano—as from anger—also comes renewal and rebirth. As the earth gives birth to itself by erupting, we can channel our anger, fear, and pain about this diagnosis into creative action and the vital will to fight.

My anger is a tool in the fight against this disease.

Shame

*I have been sick and I found out, only then,
how lonely I am. Is it too late?*

Eudora Welty

The unwarranted and confusing shame that follows a diagnosis of cancer colors our perceptions of how others see us. Since we are feeling out of control, alienated from our bodies, and no longer sure of ourselves, we expect that others are seeing us as less valuable, too.

Why jump to imaginary conclusions? Does it make sense to withdraw on the basis of how we believe others will respond to us? Withdrawal assures us of only one thing: isolation. It takes time and practice to discover who we are and the process now, as in any other time of life, means risking vulnerability.

I will not let my unexpected feelings of shame
close me off from others.

Death Sentence

The time on either side of now stands fast.
                                            Maxine Kumin

Despite our fears and suspicions, hearing the actual diagnosis of breast cancer from a doctor is always a shock. And in its wake, time stands still.

As Jory Graham pointed out in her book, *In the Company of Others*, what we hear in those first few stony seconds as time grinds to a halt is "less like a medical fact from a doctor and more like a verdict from a judge. What we hear is 'I have been sentenced to death,' and in your heart of hearts, you know that it is for a crime that you did not commit."

All we have to remember is that there is no judge and that we are the prosecution, the defense, and the jury.

A diagnosis alone does not condemn me.

Delayed Diagnosis

It is by surmounting difficulties, not by sinking under them, that we discover our fortitude.
Hannah Webster Foster

Who can know what might have been different if our physical problems had been dealt with sooner? Feel the anger. Grieve the delay. But, more importantly, this is the time to ask, what can we do about it *now*? Self-pity changes nothing. We take our anger and use it positively. It spurs us on to the next step, which is the fighting.

Starting today, I fight.

Urgency

Time . . . is so precious
that it's only given to us moment by moment.

Amelia Barr

As we grapple with this diagnosis, cancer is our new shadow, a shifting presence blurring our vision of the future. We are pulled into the present in a way we have likely never been before. A new sense of urgency takes over. But we do what we have to do, taking each moment as it comes, and that giant shadow slowly recedes.

I stay in the moment and focus on what is in front of me.

Rage

*In some ways it's my rage that keeps me going.
Without it, I would have been whipped long ago.*

Etta James

Cancer requires patience with the medical system and with the well-meaning people all around us. But the time comes when we're tired of waiting for the doctor, or for more test results. We're fed up with feeling dependent and acting brave. Out of nowhere comes an anger that fractures our self-pity. We rage against cancer and everything it has dumped in our lap. This is a bare-knuckles, "Get out of my way," "I've had enough" kind of rage.

Feel it. Express it. Sometimes it is only our anger that gets us through the day.

I acknowledge my anger at having cancer, let it out, and move on.

Isolation

To be alone is to be different;
to be different is to be alone.

Suzanne Gordon

Who around us can really understand? Do they have cancer? Are they suddenly facing death? What do they know? We ask ourselves these questions because we have the feeling of being cut off from people who haven't had to face this experience, even the people closest to us.

These feelings are natural. Breast cancer has a surreal, distancing effect. But while we are inside this shell of sorrow, we must try to avoid becoming isolated, stuck between our fate and bitterness over what has happened to us.

I leave an opening through which I can reach out to others.

Alienation

It is here that we feel . . .
a strong force from the Self, saying,
"Do not throw me away. Keep me. You'll see."
Clarissa Pinkola Estés

Does it seem easier to avoid mentioning breast cancer than to face the possible rejection inherent in letting people know? How painful a choice that is, given that our needs for communication and support are now at their greatest.

Reaching out to others is actually a way of working through feelings of alienation. It is an opportunity for those around us to demonstrate their appreciation of us, to show us that we have not changed in their eyes.

By communicating what I need, I create the possibility of getting it.

Peer Support

The burden is so heavy just now,
the task is so great . . . reinforcement is needed.
                              Mary McLeod Bethune

We're grateful for our family and friends, but it seems they have expectations of us, too. They want us to be strong, optimistic, to fight. The doctors ask us to make serious treatment choices on mastectomy, lumpectomy, reconstruction, radiation, and chemotherapy. We feel vulnerable, shifting between wanting to take charge and wanting to be told what to do. We vacillate between options and get frustrated with the uncertain outcomes.

This may be the time to reach out to other women with breast cancer who understand what it feels like when the ground under our feet disappears and we're in freefall. In a support group that's comfortable, where sharing feels safe and silence is embraced, strangers become staunch advocates and invaluable teachers. Confidence in our ability to do what we need to do grows.

I must make some hard decisions now, but I don't have to do it alone.

Respect

No one can make you feel inferior
without your consent.

Eleanor Roosevelt

It is important for our doctor-patient relationships to include respect and open communication. But how do we translate such ideal goals into the reality of a relationship that's under pressure and time constraints? How do we relate when the common perception is that we are at the mercy of the doctor (the expert) and that we must be the obedient patient, who waits in the waiting room for our turn?

Say, "It is my life at stake and I am responsible for it." When the time comes to ask questions about treatment options, perhaps even to question a point of authority or to express dissatisfaction with the level of attention we receive, do it. This is all part of the back–and–forth flow of respectful communication. This, too, is part of your healing.

I express my opinions and doubts to my doctor,
fostering respect.

Fear

Usually we think that brave people have no fear.
The truth is that they are intimate with fear.

Pema Chödrön

Brave was the last thing I felt when I found out I had cancer. After the numbness wore off, I felt only fear. As I navigated the many appointments of those early days, I saw other patients, women in various stages of treatment, coming and going with calm determination. Some were taking on the role of "pink warrior" with all their might, encouraging others. Others preferred a quiet corner and a good book. I heard laughter and that special sarcasm that comes with acting normal when we feel anything but. I saw how with each step, we move through the fear because we have no choice. Fear becomes a companion, if not a friend, and teaches us how to be brave.

In accepting my fear, I discover courage.

Self-Advocacy

That's what I like about you; you're like me.
We're both going to make it because
we're both too tough and crazy not to.

Audre Lorde

I am not a pessimist, but I don't look at the world through rose-colored glasses either. Breast cancer is hard and I decided I would be just as hard back. I'm not going to let it bring me down.

My way of staying up and moving forward is to ask questions and learn all I can about surviving this disease. I seek out other women facing breast cancer to see how they get through the tough days and long nights. Talking to them affirms my belief that while we're all determined to beat this disease, we each get to fight it in our own way.

My commitment to doing what's right for me is a powerful weapon in this fight.

Doctor–Patient Relationship

*It's a human relationship, not a
relationship between an expert and a problem.*
Rachel Naomi Remen

Many of us put on our big girl pants and started managing our health long ago. We educated ourselves and found doctors we liked. But breast cancer can intimidate even the most assertive woman. Confidence dissolves and dependency on expertise grows as we realize the complexity of this disease. There are often more questions than answers, but we can ask for what we need. If a doctor's response doesn't feel right, we can find another. We deserve a relationship based on mutual respect and trust.

&

I will find a doctor I feel comfortable with, one
who responds to my needs.

Mortality

Death, when it approaches, ought not to take one by surprise. It should be part of the full experience of life.
Muriel Spark

We're a species hardwired for survival, and denying our own end comes easily when things are good. But as the reality of cancer sets in, death is suddenly tangible in all its dimensions.

We begin to face the fact of our own death, the inevitable end to each human life. We might even make a list of all the things we're going to do before we die, things we wished we hadn't put off. We come to accept that we *will* die, maybe sooner rather than later. With this knowledge, we discover that our fear of death subsides and our appreciation for each moment grows.

I will stay in the present and not lose time to despair.

Sadness

*Perhaps we have not fully understood
that anger is a . . . cover for hurt.*

Charlotte Painter

Some days I feel a strange joy for all that I've experienced since my diagnosis, even for the difficult, for the struggles with my body and myself. Other days, while reflecting on what cancer is teaching me, I want to lash out with all my might. In spite of what I'm coming to understand at a deepening level, I'd give all my newfound insights back in a second to *not* have cancer. I'm so angry. Life may go on without me.

I try to see my illness as an opportunity, but some days I am just plain sad.

Letting Go

Letting go is knowing there is a future.
Daphne Rose Kingma

I'm a woman who likes to control things, and believe me, I have come at this disease with both barrels blasting. But I have also cried and wailed and devoted a lot of energy to letting my feelings out.

I've let go in other ways, too. I've let go of outcomes. I am fully aware that I can't control them. The only thing I can control is myself. Letting go is a way of mastering the emotional roller coaster that follows a diagnosis. It is the other side of control, and just as important as hanging on and being tough and scrappy.

Today I let go of what I can't control and discover I can master this emotional ride.

Acceptance

*In each of us there is a place we go
in the middle of chaos . . . that "home" place,
that hiding place, that soft place . . .*

Joan Chittister

We are angry, sad, and fearful that cancer happened to us. We are trying to adjust to this new reality. We may even feel guilty when we see the pain in the faces of our loved ones as they struggle with our diagnosis.

It is difficult to reassure others before we have calmed our inner turmoil. We can take the time we need to go to that quiet place inside each of us and find the peace that comes with acceptance.

I go inside myself and come to terms with my illness, easing the struggle.

Sharing the News

While all deception requires secrecy,
all secrecy is not meant to deceive.

Sissela Bok

We may need to resolve our own feelings about breast cancer before we risk sharing the news and exposing ourselves to the questioning gazes of others. It is natural to be reticent at this time, but prolonged reticence may be a signal that we need to examine our underlying fears.

It seems a fair decision if, at first, we wish to share the news with only our partner or a close friend. Still, we need to consider whether we are consciously or unconsciously locking ourselves away in a prison of silence in order to sidestep the fear of rejection—the shame-producing expectation that a cancer diagnosis has diminished us in the eyes of others. This is a natural fear, but we don't let it stop us from discovering the ones who are waiting to embrace and support us.

I will not keep my cancer a secret out of fear
or shame, but will risk sharing my news with
those who care about me.

Telling the Children

I have wept to see thee weep.
Mary Robinson

I didn't cry when the doctor told me I had breast cancer. I had prepared myself for bad news after repeated screenings and tests. When I told my husband, his shock and pain left him silent, fighting back tears, until finally, we both cried. Hardest of all, though, was telling the children. "Mom" is supposed to be there for you forever. She's supposed to be there for *your* kids someday, too.

Kids know cancer is bad. You hold them and weep together. But later, you look in their eyes and see hope. You see their belief that you will be okay, that the medicine will take care of everything, and you, too, believe.

I will be honest with my children and sustained by our mutual hope.

Self-Doubt

It is easy to relate what is of no importance.
Colette

I needed to announce the news to others, to say over and over again, "I have breast cancer." It was a way of making the news real. It was a way of integrating this devastating change, this blow to myself. Because suddenly I saw myself as different from others, as though I was marked by cancer and death. And I imagined that others saw me in the same way. But I had no frame of reference for how to best share the news. Telling others as randomly and indiscriminately as I did was not necessarily wise, but it was a psychological necessity. I had to get the words out. It was a way to dispel the shock and horror and my feelings about myself by driving them out—literally—on my breath.

I announce to others, "I have breast cancer," and wonder if I am still the same person in their eyes.

Spousal Support

Have you ever listened to two men talk? They talk about fixing things and doing things. They see the world in an active way. So my husband and I have hit upon a term that makes a lot of sense to him as a man. He is the subcontractor in my fight with this disease. His duty is to hear me rage, hear me cry, but not try and fix anything. He cannot make me well. I am in charge of that.

⁂

My husband is the "subcontractor" in my fight
with this disease. I am the contractor.

Touch

*I've learned that every day you should reach out
and touch someone. People love a warm hug,
or just a friendly pat on the back.*

Maya Angelou

When we're diagnosed with breast cancer, our initial reaction may be to withdraw from being touched, distancing ourselves from the body that has betrayed us. But there is nothing more soothing when stressed than being gently touched. Maybe it's a warm embrace, or a squeeze of the hand, but the simple act of someone reaching out and touching us is comforting.

The physical and emotional benefits of touch are well documented. With it, we calm down, blood pressure decreases, and we begin to relax. Without it, anxiety, depression, and distress can increase. A simple hug from a child, sitting close to someone who cares for us, having our hair washed, or even cuddling with a pet, are all ways of touching that can relieve our fears at this stressful time.

Touching and being touched give me strength and courage.

Faith

Many are the instruments
through which the soul seeks utterance.

Peggy Baum Gerry

I know a woman whose spiritual faith is so strong that she is able to accept whatever happens to her, even breast cancer, believing it is part of God's plan for her. I watched her respond with serenity and sincere optimism to her diagnosis. She said she would pray for me, as well as herself. I thanked her, amazed at her graciousness in the face of this cruel disease.

My faith is the wavering kind. I could never quite believe that everything happens for a reason. It would be a great comfort to believe that, especially when facing your own mortality. Letting go would come more easily, as would hope. But I accept her prayers on my behalf because I do believe that showing love and concern for another has the power to heal us both.

I find comfort in women of deep faith, as well as
in those who live with their doubts.

Optimism

*The beauty of the world has two edges, one of laughter,
one of anguish, cutting the heart asunder.*

Virginia Woolf

I've always been an optimistic person, even when bad
things happen to me. So when my doctor confirmed that
the lump I found in my breast was cancer, I went home and
researched this disease. I trust my doctor, but I want to
know what I'm up against so I can beat it.

I also read stories about strong, positive women who have
survived and I'm following their lead. There was one night,
though, when I woke up and suddenly thought to myself,
I don't want to die. The possibility hit me hard and I was
afraid. But I refuse to put myself at death's door. I focus on
getting through what is in front of me. I live my life *now*.

I feel the fear and get through the moment,
believing there are more good ones to come.

Identity

One faces the future with one's past.
Pearl S. Buck

No matter who we are and how strong we are, encountering cancer awakens all kinds of fears, threats, and anxieties. It is a threat to our life, to our sense of self, and our identity as a woman, whether we are facing mastectomy or lumpectomy.

Now is the time to strive to bring the "I" we know ourselves to be and the new "I," so recently defined by cancer, together. Absorb the knowledge of breast cancer, without letting it negate the women we know we are.

My cancer merges with everything I know to be true about me, yet it never exclusively defines me.

Information Gathering

God made the world round
so we would never be able to see too far down the road.
Isak Dinesen

We are doing the best we can in this process, at a pace we can handle. It is a fine balancing act, to gather information when each new bit stimulates new worries, and upsets the balance. The anxiety may become so intense as to temporarily cut off the desire to know. Be patient. Accept that as each piece of information hits home, it may cause another shock wave. But as the disease becomes more real, it becomes more manageable.

When the shock waves are too intense and we back off, we can congratulate ourselves for being so practical. It is the mind's way of keeping us from looking too far down the road until we recover our balance. Trust that there is an inner self that will ensure we get the information we need.

I'll put my glasses back on tomorrow when I'm again ready to see to the horizon.

Statistics

Prophecy is the most gratuitous form of error.
George Eliot

Like Benjamin Disraeli said, I now believe that there are three kinds of lies: "lies, damned lies, and statistics." We can repeat this to ourselves if we find we are sinking under the odds of beating cancer. We are vulnerable, and many of us are uninitiated in the world of statistics. But we won't let the numbers come at us as hard realities. They aren't.

Statistics are an abstraction. As the biologists tell us, variation is nature's only true essence. So while statistics talk about averages and medians, remember that each of us is a "varying" individual. We use information to inform our choices, not to stifle hope with numbers. What's most important is how we respond to our disease.

I consider the statistics and continue on my individual path.

Options

*Everything is so dangerous
that nothing is really very frightening.*

Gertrude Stein

We are confronted with a number of treatment decisions, all of which seem frightening at first. Doctors offer us a plan based on our personal situations, but there are options and it is up to us to choose. We may feel like Goldilocks, going back and forth, rejecting the ones that are too hot or too cold, trying to find the ones that are just right for us. But these are tough choices with long-term consequences. Lumpectomy or mastectomy? Chemo, radiation, or both? Reconstruction now, later, or never? Targeted post-treatment drugs and therapies or none?

Though we may feel unsure about which weapons to use, the good news is that we get to choose what's right for our fight.

I trust that I am making the best treatment choices for me.

Conflicting Opinions

I will work in my own way,
according to the light that is in me.

Lydia Maria Child

There is a divining power inside us. Focus inward. Notice fully and deeply your response to each opinion. If two opinions differ, seek a third. If one in particular makes you angry, trust that reaction.

By holding both information and emotion inside us, without striving for a resolution, we can best discover which opinion feels right. Once we've decided, we may feel anger with the doctors whose opinions we reject. It is all part of the decision-making process.

Decision-making is an opportunity to do what is right for me.

Indecision

I'm not afraid of storms,
for I'm learning how to sail my ship.

Louisa May Alcott

If we were sailing, we couldn't travel in a straight line because we'd need to capture the wind in our sails. We'd tack back and forth, zigzagging across the imaginary straight line that leads to our port. Deciding about cancer treatment is like that, too.

Lumpectomy? Mastectomy? Chemotherapy? Radiation? Reconstruction? All we can do is sail back and forth on swells of emotion and doubt, propelled forward by the force of research. As in sailing, the back-and-forth motion of making up our minds is really the only way to get the wind behind us and get where we want to go.

I allow myself the time I need to process my many decisions.

Possibilities

*The first, easiest, and most obvious assistance
toward an individual's private efforts
is the simple association with others
making the same attempt.*

Anonymous

The news kept changing from hour to hour as different tests came in. I was sinking fast. I wanted to make a plan, but my plans kept collapsing.

A woman in the doctor's office told me she was having her second mastectomy. She was undaunted, elegant. I was very impressed.

How could she be so buoyant with a double mastectomy? I wasn't willing to accept just words. I wanted to see. I asked her to show me. She agreed.

I realize now that I didn't just see a reconstructed breast; I saw a reconstructed person. She told me to never let cancer stop me. I knew what I hadn't known moments before: If it had to be a mastectomy, I could live with that, too.

I see the possibilities when I look to other women going through this.

Deciding

To have a crisis and act upon it is one thing.
To dwell in perpetual crisis is another.

Barbara Grizzuti Harrison

If we feel caught in cycles of indecision and fearfulness, we can try separating the overwhelming question before us into two threads and ask ourselves:

What is the significance of my breasts to my experience of self as a woman?

What are my attitudes toward cancer?

Then, we can try to knit these two threads back together, interweaving our feelings about cancer with the threat to our identity as women. What does the whole cloth say?

Today I consider my feelings, examine my options, and make a decision.

Intuition

*Intuition is a spiritual faculty and does not explain,
but simply points the way.*

Florence Scovel Shinn

We listen to the facts and trust our gut feelings. There is
logic, but feelings are important, too. We initiate a dialogue between head and heart in assimilating all that we
hear, remembering that it is possible for gut feelings to
change. Some of us start the process of deciding on treatment options with absolute certainty that one option, a
lumpectomy for example, is the way to go. Even in the face
of contrary medical opinions, some of us will stick to our
initial gut feelings. Some of us go back to our gut, sit with
more information, and decide that mastectomy is now our
choice. Though our hearts and minds may change in the
process of choosing treatment, trust that we will know
what is necessary and right for ourselves.

My treatment decision comes from inside me.

Confidence

It was all happening in a great, swooping free fall,
irreversible, free of decision,
in the full pull of gravity toward whatever was to be.
Laura Z. Hobson

After I anxiously awaited the news, the doctor came in and told me that my pathology report revealed lymph node involvement, my cancer was rated intermediate to high, and I would need chemotherapy. I was overwhelmed by fear and imagined the worst. So, I brought myself back to the present moment. I let myself face the facts of what I now knew; I would have chemotherapy. My fear was supplanted by acceptance and resolve—not for cancer, but for what I knew I had to do next.

I will feel the fear, face it, and do what I need to do.

Right to Choose

Where, after all, do universal human rights begin?
In small places, close to home—so close and small
that they cannot be seen on any map of the world.

Eleanor Roosevelt

We might speak as if we are making a choice, but we need to be certain that we are, indeed, the ones who made the choice. We can fall prey to making decisions that are too fast for us but the right speed for someone else. Some of us have loved ones who want the cancer out and gone and done with as fast as possible. In the pressure of the moment we might comply, see two doctors in two days, and within the week our breasts are off. We can spare ourselves the anguish of pleasing others today and then living with their decision for the rest of our lives.

We can choose to cherish what is fundamental—our rights. It is necessary to take our time, to bring our mind and body together so that we are fully prepared. That is almost more important than what we choose.

I have the right to choose my tomorrow.

Part II.

Treatment and Recovery
A Time to Heal

Paradox

*Healing is always asking us to step inside the circle,
not let going forward . . . get in the way
of being inside this moment.*

Saki Santorelli

Breast cancer is a paradox. First we're told we have it and there's nothing to do but *surrender* to this fact. Then we're told we must be strong and *fight* it, yet most of the weapons we're offered make us sick, tired, and alter our bodies as well as our very identities.

Our decisions have been made but our confidence wavers. How do we get through all that lies ahead? We take each moment as it comes, doing what we need to do—giving in and going on simultaneously.

Staying in the moment is how we move forward.

Surgery

*It appears that even the different parts of the
same person do not converse among themselves,
do not succeed in learning from each other
what are their desires and their intentions.*

Rebecca West

Surgery is a moment of truth. It brings together all the questions and doubts of different parts of who we are. If we listen as we lie in our hospital beds, we hear a disjointed conversation in our heads expressing our conflicting fears.

I fear cancer. I want it out. Surgery isn't hard. I'll be asleep. How do I live with this surgery? Can anyone tell me now, before they wheel me in, how it will change my life and my sense of self as a woman? How can I worry about that when my life is at stake? How can I live with a body that I might never love again? I'm scared.

We acknowledge the choice to undergo surgery as a step forward in the resolution of our personal crisis. We accept lumpectomy or mastectomy as the start of a transition whose outcome we cannot know. We forgive ourselves our fears and face the uncertainty with courage.

I welcome the surgery and shed tears for myself.

Private Partings

We one, must part in two . . .
                    Christina Rossetti

The night before surgery, all alone, I said goodbye to my breast. I centered myself in the hospital bed and, with my gown off, ran my hands up and down the sides of my body. It was a way to take in my body as it would be no more, intact and complete, with all its curves. My hands went around my breasts and in at the waist, out again at the hips and over my thighs.

I didn't worry about what was coming next or how I might feel the next day. I stayed right there in the moment. It was peaceful, not angry or bitter, just sad. I was saying good-bye, letting go. It was a moving parting, like an embrace you see between two people who are forced to part under duress. I was both the soldier and the bride at wartime, bidding farewell.

I say goodbye to my breast, knowing that my farewell seeds a new beginning.

The Morning After

You gave me wings to fly, then took away the sky.
Leonora Speyer

I fully expected that my surgery would go well, that it would *not* be the most momentous event in my life. I was older and married. I had already nursed and raised my kids. I thought I would be okay emotionally. But when I woke up in the hospital the day after the surgery with only one breast, I was devastated.

Who can ever accurately anticipate such feelings of loss? No one. We must enter the hospital understanding that we cannot predict what our emotions will be despite how sure we are of our treatment choices.

૭ঌ

The morning after, I acknowledge my emotions as they rise to the surface.

Walking the Hallways

People seldom see the halting and painful steps
by which the most insignificant success is achieved.
Anne Sullivan

Postsurgery hit me like a truck. Maybe it was the intravenous painkillers, or the reconstructive device inserted under my chest wall at the time of my mastectomy.

As groggy as I was, I insisted on getting up. I don't know why, but I felt as if my whole identity as a healthy woman rested on flexing my muscles and using my body immediately. Walking for me was purely a symbolic act. And the first time I tried it, it was the hardest thing I ever did.

I set a goal of walking to the end of the hallway and back. And when I got there and turned around, I thought I heard the crowds cheering. As small a victory as it was on the surface, it was a turning point for me.

I make exercise a goal to speed my emotional as well as my physical recovery.

Hospital Blues

*One reason our society has become such a mess
is that we're isolated from each other.*
                                    Maggie Kuhn

We wake up to a hospital environment away from the mainstream of our lives, far from the daily habits that define us. It is a place full of strangers, moving and acting according to a rhythm that is theirs, not ours. It is not unusual to feel alienated or lonely, intimidated or frightened. Hospital routines may infuriate us at times, too. Strange as they are, they too will become familiar and give us structure. Personalities will emerge from among the staff members and fellow patients, and our own personalities will emerge, too.

The hospital is a community and while I'm there,
I'm part of it.

Going Home

The delicate and infirm go for sympathy
not to the well and buoyant, but to those
who have suffered like themselves.
Catharine Esther Beecher

Once we are home from the hospital, the first emergency is over, or so it may seem to the people around us. But for us, the emergency has only deepened and is more fully felt. Time and space open up into loneliness and feelings of abandonment as sympathy and attention drift away. As we face further treatment, negative thoughts may also creep in: *Where is everybody? Nobody knows how I feel. How can I be so self-centered and feel forgotten by the very people who just rallied around me? Is it fair to expect any more?*

Feeling forgotten or isolated is not unusual. With everyone else caught up in the bustle of work and play, it is easy to feel left behind. Now is the time to reach out to the many other women who share our immediate needs and concerns. We can offer one another the support we need.

I reach out to other women with breast cancer to
find the support only we can offer one another.

Facing Treatment

Alone in the dark, I am going mad,
counting my sorrows.

Chu Shu-chen

We are in the dark, except for knowing that fear of the treatment has overtaken fear of the disease. It is very hard, when we feel well, to bring ourselves to choose to suffer. It is very hard, when we feel well, to choose to remove or alter our breasts. The process of choosing is a process of coming to terms with what we believe we must do. Now is the time to let it be done.

I move out of the shadows, knowing my treatment will shed light on the path I've chosen.

Courage

We are adhering to life now
with our last muscle,
the heart.

Djuna Barnes

After surgery, with its pain, dressings, drains, pills, and potential complications, we face various treatments. While some have fewer and less severe side effects, there are no easy ones. They all require stamina, and at the same time, sap our strength. Radiation is its own invisible form of hell-fire. And the chemicals in chemotherapy, when spilled, are handled as hazardous waste with protective clothing, gloves, and masks.

When we're feeling overwhelmed by what comes next, we take heart. Simply holding on and hanging in there is its own kind of courage, and one that serves us well as we face new challenges ahead.

Today I find the courage to take on treatment.

Focus

One never notices what has been done;
one can only see what remains to be done . . .

Marie Curie

We pride ourselves on being multitaskers and superwomen when it comes to juggling our responsibilities. Some of us charge into treatment, convinced we can handle a little nausea and fatigue and still do it all. We know about doing it all, eating on the run, working late, and taking care of others.

With weeks and months of treatment ahead, it is time to focus on ourselves and practice the healing art of saying "no" to the demands of daily life as often as we say "yes."

My focus turns to me as I go through treatment.

Prayer

We acknowledge a larger reality
when we pray, however we pray,
that reality is essentially something mysterious.
Rachel Naomi Remen

For those who seek rational answers to life's questions, breast cancer is a challenge. We accept the diagnosis, research our options, and go forward, sticking to the facts. But as we face treatment we realize that while we better understand the disease, we are still asking, "Why me?"

This may be a question without an answer, but one worth praying about. Prayer connects us to something greater than ourselves, whether that is God, Mother Earth, the Great Spirit, or the universe of other human beings who are suffering and wondering. Prayer is a way to acknowledge that we don't have all the answers and we don't need to in order to live through and beyond this reality.

Prayer is my way of living with the questions.

Radiation

*This cancer business was an emergency
for which I had to gather all my forces.*
                        Mary Roberts Rinehart

Some say the process of receiving radiation treatment is easier than that of chemotherapy. But radiation treatment is a tough commitment, too. We live with it intimately, showing up for treatment five days a week for up to six weeks. And some effects are permanent, such as a tightening of the connective tissue on the chest wall, a condition that does not fade away like transitory symptoms of fatigue and nausea. But first and foremost, radiation is a commitment to well-being.

☙

I gather my forces to do what I believe will make me well.

Shared Effort

*Then give to the world the best you have,
and the best will come back to you.*

Madeline Bridges

Radiation treatments are a daily reminder of cancer. I felt I couldn't get away from this disease, when every day radiation summoned me backward instead of on with life. But gradually, I started to open up. I started to see another side. I began to recognize the faces and the stories of the other women who received regular treatments alongside me. I got to know the doctors and the nurses and staff. I focused on these relationships and how they grew over the days and weeks. I came to see my treatments as a daily, shared effort toward my healing.

I open up to the supportive relationships all around me in my daily treatments.

First Cycle of Chemo

Necessity is also an object of exploration.
Simone Weil

The first cycle of chemotherapy treatment is the hardest, going through it as we are by necessity and not knowing what to expect. Desperate questions such as "What is it like?" and "What can I do about the side effects?" go unanswered until the first direct experience.

With the first treatment behind us, however, we can experiment. A good place to start is to monitor how we're feeling and consider what might be the best time of day for infusion or taking our drugs. And working with our oncology team, we can monitor our response to the anti-anxiety and anti-nausea medicines. Staff members can also advise us on the right foods to eat, and what to avoid, before and after treatment as well as between treatments to maximize appetite and nutrition. Some side effects are inevitable, but we can explore all the ways to minimize the worst symptoms and get through each cycle successfully.

I explore ways to meet the treatment commitment I have made.

Visualization

Woes have their ebb as well as their flow.
Katherine Fowler Philips

After the needle has gone in for the chemical infusion, ask for a blanket. Bundle up and begin:

Start with the toes. Focus on them and relax them. Next, your feet, ankles, calves, thighs, all the way up to your head. When your body is still, take it on a relaxation journey.

Visualize a big dark sky, and way out there in the distance a yellow blinking light.

Focus on the light, and as it gets nearer, see that it says "relax." Watch as the word gently pulses, dimming and brightening. Watch the pulsing yellow light as it transmutes into a golden sun above a white sand beach. See yourself, stretched out there. Let the sand contour to your body. Listen to the waves and let the sun warm you. Feel how that warmth becomes one with the elixir of treatment. Imagine how the sunlight and elixir together move through your body, eliminating cancer cells and warming you into a state of relaxed and satisfying sleep.

I create my own healing environment during treatment.

Hope

*Hope is the feeling you have
that the feeling you have isn't permanent.*

Jean Kerr

Every time we're hit with chemotherapy we see ourselves being dropped down a dark hole. And then we see ourselves working our way back to the top. But just as we get to the top, someone steps on our fingers—we are given another treatment—and down we go again. We can't minimize the falling down part. It's real. But we like to focus on the climbing back up, on all the creative ways we can work our way back to the top.

♡

Today I discover new ways to climb out of the dark hole of treatment and back up to the top.

Exercise

I can remember walking as a child.
It was not customary to say you were fatigued.
It was customary to complete
the goal of the expedition.

Katharine Hepburn

Despite the chemotherapy, we incorporate exercise into our routine. Exercise helps us sleep, helps combat the depression from the chemotherapy, and the depression from what we're going through. We see exercise as a way to fight the cancer. Sometimes it's hard, but afterwards we feel vibrant and alive and a healthy kind of tired, not the fatigue of chemotherapy. Our body feels stronger and meeting our personal exercise goals is good for our self-esteem at this vulnerable moment in our life.

Today I will do whatever I can to move my body.

Sharing Our Story

Sisters: talk to each other . . . share your stories.
Together we are invincible.

Isabel Allende

Not all of us are comfortable in a support group. We're reluctant to talk about ourselves, and we may resist anything—group support, group hugs, group walks, and pink ribbons—that identifies us as "a woman with breast cancer."

We don't have to become somebody we are not. But we reap powerful emotional benefits when we have someone to talk to, someone who listens, cares, and keeps our confidences. It might be a sister, a close friend, or someone you met in a group who also seems to be quietly hanging back. There are people waiting to help us carry our burdens, to help us heal in a way that works for us.

⁓

Sharing my story with a trusted listener lightens my load.

Healing Ritual

We must humbly pray to the rocks,
the trees, the sky . . . to help us
with all our struggles . . . and help us to heal.

International Council
of Thirteen Indigenous Grandmothers

Each time I came home from a round of chemo, I felt relief at putting one more infusion behind me, but also terror that the drugs' dire side effects were manifesting. With months of treatment ahead, I decided to mark the passage of time in a way that would soothe and sustain me.

I had a collection of rocks—small, large, pretty, and plain ones—picked up over the years on close-to-home walks and faraway treks. I selected a rock for each remaining infusion and put them into one bowl, then placed an empty bowl beside it. After each treatment, I picked up a rock from the first bowl, held it a moment, and placed it in the second bowl saying, "I can do this." Watching that second bowl fill up reinforced my commitment to chemotherapy and brought peace in the midst of distress.

❧

I nurture my healing through simple acts that
sustain my courage.

Hair Loss

Love is a great beautifier.
                              Louisa May Alcott

When I lost my hair to chemotherapy and became bald, I was like Samson. Somehow, all my self-worth and emotional strength seemed to be rooted in my scalp. I broke down and grieved in the way you might grieve over the loss of someone you love. My husband took me by the shoulders and said, "Look at me. I'm the man that you love and I'm bald."

He was right. So what if I'm bald? So is he. And my hair is going to grow back, which is more than he can say. I love him anyway. He is wonderful in my eyes, and realizing that, I know I am still beautiful to him.

Today I make a list of all the people without hair who I love and put my name at the top.

Infertility

Leaving aside the bough that produced beauty's fruit,
Inclining toward a bough that no such fruit does show.
Wallada

As premenopausal women facing chemotherapy, what crashes in on us is the temporary, if not the permanent, loss of fertility brought on by treatment. Whether we plan to bear children or already have a house full of them, loss of fertility is still a cut to the fabric in which we, as women, cloak ourselves.

Feminine identity is woven from many things, including fertility and the possibility of giving birth. Yet being female transcends fertility and breasts; it is an essence that cannot be lost.

～

Today I celebrate myself as a woman of courage and possibility.

Working

*The idea of strictly minding our own business
is moldy rubbish. Who could be so selfish?*
Myrtie Lillian Barker

I never hid from my coworkers the fact of my cancer or that I was undergoing treatment. That was my choice, my particular solution. My world had gone crazy, but I needed to work and I didn't want to hide.

There is a benefit in being so forthright. I found out that everyone I know professionally has had some contact with breast cancer, either directly or through a friend of a friend. I didn't feel isolated among them. They were interested, supportive, concerned. Many were educated by my experience. They went out and had their own breasts checked, or urged their wives, partners, and family members to do so. Coworkers are professional colleagues, but they are also human beings.

⁊

I share my breast cancer experience and my
relationships deepen, even my professional ones.

Depression

Clouds behind clouds in long succession rise . . .
Anna Letitia Barbauld

Many of us experience an organic depression during che-motherapy, a depression that goes well beyond any we might already be feeling. It is not the sort of depression that we can will ourselves out of. The cloud of depression that follows treatment is a physiological response, not an emo-tional one.

This depression is physical, so much so that some days we don't want to get up, as though depression has gotten into our bones. It's easy to blame ourselves for how we feel, but we can blame the drugs! And we can remind ourselves that we are "in the chemo."

We find solace knowing in advance that a few days later the depression will pass like a cloud. We wait and notice when it lifts. Suddenly we feel alive again.

I know that these treatment blues will, like the clouds, soon pass.

Sisters

For there is no friend like a sister
In calm or stormy weather . . .
                              Christina Rossetti

I always try to be there for my younger sister, so I felt a little guilty when *I* was the one who needed help. As sisters, we've been through more than a few ups and downs together, and we've seen each other at our best and our worst. Maybe that's why her unwavering support during my treatment was so comfortable and easy to accept.

She was there for me from the start, rearranging her life, bringing her child and dogs and music to my home, flushing my chest catheter, cooking dinner, making me laugh, and being who she is—the light of my world.

I am forever grateful for the loving support that only a sister-friend can give.

The Comfort of Friends

Best friend, my well-spring in the wilderness . . .
George Eliot

It is only very, very good friends that I consent to see in the few days directly after treatment. When I can't trust myself to be myself, I need blind faith in the people I have around me. I feel like a wild animal, yet I hope for caring, compassion, and understanding. I want comfort. I want to be an unabashed bumbling idiot, yet feel myself still loved.

And my friends not only bring me comfort, but they give my family some relief from the stress of caregiving. My friends' willingness to be with me under these conditions is a show of support. I accept their gift as a wonderful statement of caring.

I am grateful for the healing power of friendship.

Restlessness and Irritability

The thing that is really hard, and really amazing,
is giving up on being perfect.

Anna Quindlen

At times, we may think we need to ask forgiveness for being ourselves, on those days when we snap, are irritable and restless, and could jump out of our skins except that we're too tired to move.

We read, take a walk, meditate, or try to stay busy with small tasks. But restlessness and irritability resurface. We lose ourselves in our favorite social media sites, an activity that quickly moves and changes, mirroring our own restlessness. But that doesn't work either.

Maybe the only way to get through these periods is as an anxious couch potato, watching television. It's okay. It happens. We remind ourselves that it's the treatments, not us, and that it's fine to ask our doctors for something to alleviate these symptoms when our usual remedies aren't working.

I forgive myself when my treatments cause me
to be restless and irritable.

Post-Treatment Support

Concern should drive us into action,
not into a depression.

Karen Horney

We celebrate the end of treatment. But a small voice, one we can hardly believe we hear, talks to us in fearful moments. *I am left on my own,* it says. *I don't see the doctor again for months. I should be happy. Why am I so anxious and scared?*

We feel a sense of connectedness and hope in the process of receiving treatment, as tough as it may be. Conversely, there is a loss in its completion. We are cut off from our doctor and our oncology team, and we are momentarily frightened in the face of the unknown. We are alone again.

We recognize this as another transition in the cancer journey. Again, it's time to move on. We allow ourselves the time it takes. We remind ourselves that our doctor is always there and we can call if we need to. We ease into it, gaining confidence with each step. And we reach out for support from other women who are on this journey with us, making new connections and renewing hope along the way.

I answer the little voice of fear I hear at the end
of treatment with patience and hope.

Healing Alternatives

Healing depends on listening with the inner ear . . .
Marion Woodman

At the beginning of this journey, we turn ourselves over to doctors, stepping onto the straightforward path of medical intervention. It is a hands-on affair, much of it hurts, and it is necessary. Now, we may want to explore alternative paths to enhance our healing, from acupuncture and massage to meditation and yoga.

Integrating alternative methods is not a rejection of traditional care, but a way to embrace the healing power within us. We give ourselves the time to sit quietly, to listen to our heart, and to explore not only the body's distress but the wounded places in mind and spirit. We begin to explore what feels right to us now, and what doesn't. We begin to heal our whole self.

I explore different ways that healing can happen
in body, mind, and spirit.

Reconstruction

*One never discusses anything with anybody
who can understand; one discusses things
with people who cannot understand.*

Gertrude Stein

Many women report that their partners discourage them
from elective reconstructive surgery out of a kind of loving protectiveness. We can appreciate those feelings, but
it's important to recognize that it's hard for anyone else to
measure the psychological necessity of such a surgery for
us. We are the only ones who know our internal pressure to
restore feelings of wholeness in terms of breast symmetry.
When considering reconstructive surgery, we need to weigh
the pros and cons and make the decision for and about ourselves, not for our partners, or anyone else in our lives.

My decision about reconstruction is up to me.

Matching Breasts

However, one cannot put a quart in a pint cup.
Charlotte Perkins Gilman

I am a large-breasted woman, and in an ideal world I would want my reconstructed breast to be the same size. But I am unwilling to reduce my remaining, healthy breast in any way for purposes of symmetrical reconstruction. I can't see afflicting my one good breast with cuts or changes. I want to preserve it, as is, a kind of monument to what was.

My breasts are an important part of my sexual pleasure and I refuse to give up my sensitivity. And I plan to have children and breastfeed them, so how can I start reducing and moving things around? For me, the current and potential functions of my remaining breast far outweigh the visual considerations of matching breasts. I know I'm going to be lopsided and I can live with that.

Breast symmetry is important to me, but it is not my primary concern.

Adjustment

A story of despair imprints the leaf.
Charlotte Elizabeth Tonna

As a woman who began the process of immediate reconstruction at the time of my mastectomy, I felt that my identity as a woman now rested on the outcome of the surgery. I was fine as long as there was hope and anticipation. But when I was faced with the results, the realization of what I had really lost washed over me.

Suddenly, I had to adjust to the differences between my two breasts. They were nothing alike, or so it seemed to me, and I got very depressed. We must prepare ourselves for a period of adjustment once reconstruction is done, particularly for those of us who go right from mastectomy to reconstruction. I had no idea there would be such a delayed reaction to the loss of my real breast, but it hit me like a ton of bricks.

I accept that adjusting comes with each step of this journey.

Satisfaction

*There must be acceptance, and the knowledge
that sorrow fully accepted brings its own gifts . . .*
                                    Pearl S. Buck

My new breast is a nice one. It was supposed to look like a
teardrop or a croissant, like my natural breast, but it ended
up looking like a grapefruit. Frankly, I don't care what kind
of breakfast food it is, as long as I have it under my skin. It
fills out my bra without me having to think about it, and on
a basic level, it gets the job done.

I miss my own breast but I am here, taking joy
in all my imperfections.

Disappointment

It is not fair to ask of others
what you are not willing to do for yourself.
Eleanor Roosevelt

I was very disappointed by my breast reconstruction. Despite all the warnings, I expected too much. I had hoped that the surgery would get me back to being natural looking. But when it was done, I realized that I wasn't anywhere near looking natural and I was never going to be. I thought that reconstruction would be the entire solution to rebuilding my self-image and that I would have little responsibility in the matter. But I was wrong. Reconstruction only lays the groundwork. I have a big part to play.

Reconstruction is only a beginning point in the process of accepting my new body.

Cleavage

Imagination has always had powers of resurrection that no science can match.

Ingrid Bengis

It has been nine years of hell and now I have had my reconstruction. Finally! After living for years with an awful flatness, all I wanted was cleavage. Period.

I am a 1950s woman. I wanted great cleavage and I got it. I think every woman should be concerned with only those illusions that mean something to her.

When I ask a doctor to sculpt my image, I have him or her do it after my own ideal.

Nipples

*What really matters is
what you do with what you have.*

Shirley Lord

My reconstructed nipple is kind of like a glass eye. It doesn't do much but sit there and fill in the blank space so I don't worry myself, or others, that something is missing. The main advantage is that when I'm nude, I don't feel like I'm "winking" at my partner anymore. He does keep asking me, over and over, if I'm sure I can't feel anything in the fake nipple. Of course I can't, but it's nice to pretend.

My fake nipple is like icing on a cake; it's not necessary, but it's a nice finishing touch.

Bonding with My Body

I am no longer what I was.
I will remain what I became.

Coco Chanel

I had to massage my new breast morning and night to keep scar tissue from forming and causing my breast to harden. At first I resented it. I wanted my breast to just "be." I didn't want to have to work at it. I didn't want the constant reminder that there was this foreign object living under my skin.

To my surprise, the daily massage caused a kind of bonding to take place. It helped me to get to know and accept my new breast. I learned the limits of my sensitivity—the beginning and end points of feeling at the perimeter of my reconstructed breast and the areas of total numbness. I learned that my breast was made of tough stuff and that I didn't have to be afraid of it. I found out it gets cold to the touch. I felt how when my chest muscles tighten over the implant, massage makes it relax. Most important of all, I learned that my reconstructed breast is a part of me.

I massage my reconstructed breast as a way of making it part of me.

Self-Pity

Life does not accommodate you,
it shatters you . . . every seed destroys its container
or else there would be no fruition.
                                        Florida Scott-Maxwell

Finally, it's over, we think to ourselves when treatment is finished, hair grows back, or reconstruction surgery is done. We tell ourselves we will put breast cancer behind us and begin again. But self-pity creeps in, clouding the future. Breast cancer breaks us open and a sense of loss can linger. In spite of our outer optimism, deep inside we may feel damaged. But beneath the hurt, our new life is waiting to emerge. Dig for it, and let it grow.

I stop feeding the pain and start nurturing the possibilities.

Self-Rejection

*When one is a stranger to oneself
then one is estranged from others too.*

Anne Morrow Lindbergh

It is natural to have feelings of fear and self-rejection as we get to know our altered bodies and altered selves. What is important is to not defend too long against those feelings because at some point, avoidance becomes a form of denial.

To really look at ourselves, inside and out, is a courageous act. Difficult as it is, it is the beginning point, the first step in the process of self-healing.

I accept my fear and confront the stranger I have become to myself.

Mirror Gazing

The work of healing is in peeling away the barriers
of fear and past conditioning that keep us unaware
of our true nature of wholeness and love.

Joan Borysenko

I set up a program. Every day I spent about fifteen minutes looking in the mirror. It was one aspect of rebuilding my body image. It was like getting to know a new friend. I approached myself openly, honestly, and with love, I made daily visual and physical contact with myself through the reflection in the mirror. Sometimes I just looked. Sometimes I talked out loud to myself. Sometimes I rubbed cream on my scar, or touched the area around it. Sometimes I tried on clothes to see how they looked—to see what worked and what didn't. Gradually I came to know, recognize, accept, and love myself once again. It did not happen overnight. But then, what long-lasting relationship does?

I look in the mirror and I say with love, "That is me. I am no better or no worse than before. It is just me."

Living with Our Choices

*I think I must be the tree but also the hole in it
pecked out by a sharp beak.
Or am I the heart, which lives in the tree?*

Deena Metzger

I told the doctor I wanted the cancer gone. "Take it out now. No half measures please, go all the way, both breasts." I was so sure that my life depended on it. Now, I am glad to be alive and feeling good. The empty space where my breasts used to be reminds me of that urgent plea to go all the way. Maybe I could have chosen differently. But I always knew I was more than my body. I love it and try to take good care of it, but in the end, it is only the container for the woman I am and the one I will become.

I make room in my heart to love my body, no matter what, as it carries me through this life.

Clothing

Dress to please yourself . . .
Forget "you are what you wear" . . .
wear what you are.

Elizabeth Hawkes

Clothing became a bigger issue for me than I ever expected. Besides the weight gain, my first prosthesis was not exactly a match for my remaining breast. I soon discovered that old wardrobe favorites—knits, t-shirts, and v-necks—revealed the imbalance. I became self-conscious about my appearance in a way I'd never been before. I spent months, and too much money, on every kind of prosthesis and bra and outfit to try and create that perfect fit.

After a long and frustrating search for perfection, I took a long look in the mirror. Yes, I had changed, and I decided that my clothes fit the woman I am now just fine.

I discover I need a change of heart more than a change of clothes.

Joy

People need joy quite as much as clothing.
Some of them need it far more.

Margaret Collier Graham

Following my mastectomy, I purchased one plain, inexpensive prosthesis bra. I only bought one because I thought I wouldn't live long enough to need another.

At a support group meeting, I noticed a bit of lace on another woman's bra. She said she had a prosthesis in it and I was absolutely stunned.

This little encounter taught me that it's not so much what happens to us but how we respond to it that reveals how we are feeling about ourselves. That woman with the lace had been through exactly what I had been through, but she dressed herself with joy.

I deserve to dress my one breast, and myself, in lace and in joy.

Show and Tell

Your audience gives you everything you need.

Fanny Brice

I had a little "show and tell" with a friend. She said she liked the way I looked better than the way she looked. That completely shocked me. Up until that point I thought of myself as disfigured, damaged, and reworked, all negative images. This friend keeps herself in shape. She dislikes the saggy stuff that is the reality of women's breasts, as we grow older. Leave it to her, a woman with two healthy breasts, to find my fake versions preferable to the real thing. Suddenly, I was upright, firm, and forever young, at least from my neck to my navel. Her perspective gave me a new way of looking at myself.

I listen to the perspectives of others to help me reaffirm my self-image.

Loss

You must do the thing you think you cannot do.
Eleanor Roosevelt

Back when I had breasts, I thought I had a nice pair. I didn't worry too much that one was a little bigger than the other, and I tried not to compare myself to other women. But now that I've lost mine, I see breasts on display everywhere. I can't imagine how I'm going to live without my real, imperfect breasts that moved when I moved, and grew old along with me. I see young women, old women, overweight, skinny, and average women, with breasts of all shapes and sizes peeking over the top, spilling out the side, or hanging down in front and I think, *How beautiful, how individual, how perfect.*

I accept my treatment choice as right for me,
and I accept the loss.

Doubt

*What happens to us becomes a part of us
in both body and mind.*

Siri Hustvedt

I kept telling myself that I *had* breast cancer, though I knew recurrence was a possibility.

I told myself that I *survived* breast cancer, past tense, and refused to call myself a *survivor.* I am *me* again, a healthy, intrepid woman who's been treated and released.

It has taken me months to realize that my attitude may not be an exercise in positive thinking, but a denial of the impact cancer has had on my mind, as well as my body. I accept the physical changes, but it is taking much longer to come to terms with the undercurrent of doubt and fear running below the surface of my confident appearance.

My well-being depends on healing my whole self, body and mind.

Self-Image

Being preoccupied with our self-image
is like . . . standing in the middle of a vast field
of wildflowers with a black hood over our heads.

Pema Chödrön

Our bodies are changed after treatment for breast cancer and we may have trouble looking in the mirror post-lumpectomy or post-mastectomy and seeing anything but a shadow of who we were.

Now is the time to look without judgment at the things that make us the unique person we are: our eyes, our smile, our arms, hands, and legs, our scars, our courage, our survival.

Like wildflowers, beauty comes in many colors, shapes, sizes, and seasons, and it blooms in the most amazing places.

I see myself as I am, full of beauty and life.

Self-Love

*The first problem for all of us, men and women,
is not to learn, but to unlearn.*

Gloria Steinem

When I first learned I had breast cancer, I heard the word
"cancer" more loudly than I heard the word "breast." I got
busy and fought the cancer. It wasn't until after treatment
that I heard the word "breast" ringing in my ears. Now I
only had one. A woman is supposed to have two. They're
a measure of her appeal, her worthiness, her power to get
what she wants.

These ideas kept running through my head, ideas I had
rejected long ago as artifacts of another time. Why did I
believe them now? I told myself I was still the same woman.
But was I? Once again, I had to let go of the belief that I was
only as good as my body looked and learn to love me, inside
and out.

I reject the idea that I am now less of a *woman*,
and discover more about the *person* I am.

Nudity

I will look for beauty today in myself . . . and find it.
                                                              Karen Casey

I believe that the physical beauty of a woman is not limited to the perfection or imperfection of her face or body.
It is how her face and body are enlivened by her spirit that
makes her beautiful. It wasn't hard for me to be nude after
my mastectomy. My scars were visual images of what I had
been through, and survived. My scars were a badge of courage and a symbol of the empathy I feel for any woman who
has to go through this.

When I stand in the nude, I want others to see
courage and empathy, which make me beautiful.

Adaptability

*Life is about not knowing, having to change,
taking the moment and making the best of it.*

Gilda Radner

Often it is when we feel the most vulnerable that we are hardest on ourselves, and the people around us. When we are angry at fate, God, or the world for what has happened to us, defenses go up and survival instincts kick in. We will not surrender. We will fight and win.

A fighter's stance is good when we first confront breast cancer. We put our bodies through nasty stuff to get better. We may find ourselves taking drugs that target our particular kind of breast cancer for years to come. But we do not have to let the fight harden our hearts. Our vulnerability gave rise to formidable courage and resilience, as we looked death in the face. It is time to make peace with this path leading us in new directions.

I am learning how to bend, not break, as I face new challenges.

Intention

The biggest sin is sitting on your ass.
Florynce R. Kennedy

Intention is a powerful tool. It is how we articulate and create what we want. If we *intend* to improve our feelings of self-worth after the changes wrought by breast cancer, we are taking responsibility. Regardless of the specific actions we take, assuming responsibility goes a long way. It is an antidote to feelings of powerlessness and of anger at ourselves and the world.

Intentions come in many forms: joining a new support group, exposing our body to a friend or loved one, pursuing breast reconstruction surgery, or tattooing over a mastectomy scar. From the cautious to the outrageous, the underlying message is that we are intending to grab our insecurities by the horns and wrestle them to the ground as deliberately as we can.

My intention is to move out of my safe zone and take action in a way that works for me.

Opening Up

Use your words.

Anonymous

Once treatment is behind us, it's nice to believe that life will go on as before. We pick up where we left off, but soon discover uncertainty gnawing at us. Every little pain is a recurrence. Every checkup is an ordeal. We can't talk to family and friends about it because they don't *really* understand what we've been through. We're feeling sorry for ourselves, again.

It's important to tell people how we're feeling, to let them know that we're doing well, but we have our moments when a little reassurance is in order. They can't read our minds, but they will understand what's going on in our hearts if we open up to them. You never know—they may be worrying, too.

I will ask for what I need, and I will ask others to do the same.

Guilt

. . . the silent deep abode of guilt.
                    Mercy Otis Warren

The women we encounter along the way are some of the most positive aspects of this experience, yet breast cancer is a very individual disease. Guilt comes with being incredibly "lucky" and bypassing tough treatments that others couldn't, or with getting through treatment with fewer side effects. The guilt is even worse when someone we care about does not respond to treatment. We're doing well and feeling guilty when they're not. But none of us can trade places, and our mutual support becomes a double-edged sword in this battle.

∾

I channel feelings of guilt into celebrating life on behalf of myself and others.

Changing Relationships

*Things falling apart is a kind of testing
and also a kind of healing.*

Pema Chödrön

We may hear the cliché about "never getting more than we can handle" from family, friends, and caregivers, and while this doesn't necessarily help, we accept their good intentions.

Cancer, like other life crises, strains relationships in predictable, as well as unexpected, ways. We may discover that a longtime relationship quietly fades into the distance. We may also discover that an acquaintance has become a valued friend. Try to remain open to the ebb and flow of support and avoidance from the people around you. Consider what's helping, and what's not. To wonder whether to let go of a relationship or hang on to it is not a test, but an opportunity for healing.

I will keep the focus on healing as cancer tests me and my relationships.

Men and Emotions

*Men have been expected to tell the truth about facts,
not about feelings. They have not been expected
to talk about feelings at all.*

Adrienne Rich

It takes time to transition from breast cancer patient to a new sense of self after diagnosis and treatment. Renewing our connection to our lover or spouse takes time, too.

In the midst of the initial crisis, many men provide support by doing things, like driving us to the doctor's office, taking care of kids and home, calling family and friends, and by just being there for us. But when we ask them to *tell* us how they're doing, they don't necessarily come through.

Try not to mistake a man's inability to communicate his feelings for a lack of love, or concern. He may be more comfortable showing us, not telling us, how he's feeling as he navigates his own transition.

We have a right to expect emotional support, but
it may come through actions, not words.

Extended Family

Quite nice women suddenly have to wear this title with the stigma on it and a crown of thorns.
Sylvia Ashton-Warner

I attended an extended family gathering. It felt like a gathering for the explicit purpose of staring at *Katy, who has breast cancer.* After an hour of it, I think most people there realized I was the same me. I don't think *I* had any doubts, but they obviously did. Let me caution all of us who go and visit family and friends; we don't have to just sit there and "have cancer." Wherever we go, we can be ourselves. Then everyone will know that cancer is not who we are; it is only one more experience we're having in life.

I send a clear message in everything I do; I am still me.

Indifference

*A woman has got to love a bad man once or twice
in her life, to be thankful for a good one.*
Marjorie Kinnan Rawlings

I look back on my marriage vows and think what a hopeless romantic I was. You can't envision "in sickness and in health, until death us do part" when you're young.

My husband was there for me during the surgeries and chemo. The next year, he left.

I now realize that he wasn't really there for me. He was just going through the motions, like he'd been doing for a long time. It took breast cancer to teach me that his silent indifference was its own kind of emotional abuse. I will not put up with that ever again.

I seek relationships that are alive and mutually supportive.

Pity

Pity is the deadliest feeling that can be offered . . .
                                        Vicki Baum

News had spread among friends and colleagues that I had breast cancer. One night at a party, my husband was solemnly asked by a man we both knew, "How is she doing?"

"She's right here," my husband said. "Ask her yourself." The look on that guy's face was clearly one of shock, pity, and embarrassment. He assumed, like so many, that you get cancer and then you die. It was the first time I realized that people would react that way to me. I didn't feel bad about it, but I was mad. I told him, "I'm fine, and I'm the same person I always was."

I reject other people's pity as a way of showing them that I am not a victim.

Solitude

*This is also a time to offer everything we know up to
the great mystery so that we might be transformed.*

Deena Metzger

Our journey through breast cancer may bring into question
the notion that we're in this together. Two people can care
for each other very much and yet be blind and deaf to each
other's perspectives, in spite of our best efforts to communicate. Filtered by distinct personalities and experiences,
the world may look very different to each of us. Grappling
with our questions and fears, one may feel optimistic while
another feels hopeless.

When we lose confidence in words, we can sit quietly with
ourselves. When we do, we are not giving up on our relationships, but turning over our need to make others see
things as we do, accepting that there are some paths that
change us so deeply that we must walk them alone.

When words fail, silence offers me comfort and
direction.

Untended Issues

Each day, we must learn again how to love . . .
                                                    Barbara Crooker

If we're lucky, we go through treatment surrounded by people who love and support us. If we're lucky, our most important relationships survive the trauma of our illness, none the worse for wear. Some of us aren't that lucky.

Even long-term relationships are tested when we confront breast cancer. We're intimate with our own fear and anger, but others don't always share what they're feeling. As we go through the ups and downs of recovery, we accept the awkward conversations that soon turn into uncomfortable silences. One day we realize that untended issues already stressing a relationship are now enough to break it. We let it go, and tend to the ones still by our side, not giving up on love.

֍

I accept that breast cancer can make or break relationships.

Gratitude

. . . Help us find the courage
To make our lives a blessing
And let us say, Amen . . .

Mi Sheberach
(Jewish prayer for healing,
Debbie Friedman, translator)

Suffering does not make us prophets or saints. It does not necessarily make us wiser, kinder, or more spiritual. It *does* remind us that no one has all the answers, or so much influence, power, or money that they don't need a little help sometimes.

Now that we're back on our feet, let us not forget the many, small acts of kindness by family and friends that brought light to a dark time. Let us remember the strangers who cared for us in extraordinary ways throughout our treatments. And let us find a way to give something back in the course of our, once again, blessed, ordinary days.

I am grateful for the help I received, and I pass it on.

Expectations

I must reluctantly admit that I am not quite as I was.
Eleanor Roosevelt

With the loss of a breast, you mourn the loss of an extremely sensitive erogenous zone.

In very real terms, you miss the lost or altered breast because it was an irreplaceable source of pleasure that is gone, or at least no longer the same. It is better to mourn your loss than to suppress those feelings.

At the same time that you acknowledge the loss is real, don't overlook the possibilities in the present. There is a healing tenderness to be found in lovemaking. Do not reject sex out of fear that the experience of it today will not match all the memories of lovemaking in the past. Your desires, hopes, and expectations are here now, waiting to be realized.

I enjoy the pleasures my body still offers me,
even as I remember what once was.

Self-Acceptance

Each day comes bearing its own gifts.
Untie the ribbons.

Ruth Ann Schabacker

Self-acceptance is the first step on the road to loving ourselves. And loving ourselves—the good, the bad, and the average—is the first step to true intimacy with a loving partner. Before breast cancer, many of us had stopped playing hide and seek in the bedroom. We knew that lovemaking was not about the joining of two perfect bodies, but about the meeting of two open hearts.

After breast cancer, that easy comfort between us and our spouses or lovers can disappear for a while. Accepting the changes to our bodies and our sexual selves takes time. Once again, we learn how to stop hiding as we seek the gift of loving intimacy.

I will share myself openly, creating an opportunity for true intimacy.

Intimacy

Those who have taken the terrible risk of intimacy . . .
know life without intimacy to be impossible.
Carolyn Heilbrun

Intimacy is an emotional and physical closeness that transcends the sexual. Even when it is expressed in sexual terms, it is not limited to the act of intercourse. Massage, hugging, kissing, touching, stroking, locking hands, sitting or sleeping together, embracing, and gazing into each other's eyes are also forms of intimacy. But the single most important element in intimacy, especially after breast cancer, may be the intimacy of dialogue.

The chief barriers now for many of us, and our partners, are fear and insecurity. Giving voice to our feelings is the only way to resolve them. Sharing our most vulnerable selves and asking for what we want, or voicing what we don't want, is at the core of an intimate relationship between any two people, whether long-married, newly dating, or anywhere in between.

Today I risk sharing my inner self.

Communication

To live in dialogue with another is to live twice.
Joys are doubled by exchange
and burdens are cut in half.

Wishart

How do we build a bridge between our altered bodies and altered self-esteem and the sexual realm? We may feel paralyzed by what has been taken from us—ways of being, doing, and looking, still fresh in our memory. How do we set aside the images of what is versus what is gone?

The answer is communication—speaking with courage and sharing needs. "Don't touch me there just now, it's too soon." Or, "Please do touch my scar, it needs love, too." Or even, "I feel so ugly," if that is how we feel at the moment. It is only by expressing such feelings that we have any hope of receiving the warmth of a healing response, the "You look beautiful to me," that each of us needs to hear.

Today I share what feels good and right, or wrong and not right, about me with my lover.

First Lovemaking

If you have a body in which you were born to a certain
amount of pain . . . why should you not,
when the occasion presents, draw from this
same body the maximum of pleasure?

Isadora Duncan

As we carry our anxieties about body image and desirability into bed with us, remember that our minds always were and always will be the final arbiter of any sexual experience. Initially, bittersweet associations are bound to well up: *My scars can be felt. My chest wall is numb. I'm out of balance.* We can stay with these thoughts and feelings as we cry the inevitable tears that come with the first sexual experience of an altered body. We can gently remind ourselves that we need and deserve the pleasurable sensations that are about to follow.

We move from emotional pain into the comfort of physical pleasure by putting aside all thoughts and letting the impact of another's touches build. Receive them as gestures of pure healing and acceptance.

I relax into my body and experience the sensual
pleasure it gives me.

Lack of Desire

*Not always the fanciest cake that's there
is the best cake to eat.*

Margaret Sanger

There is definitely sex after breast cancer if we define sex as everything we do with our partners, from cuddling to simply sleeping next to one another. Yes, the aftereffects of treatment are still there and some of us may have descended into premature menopause. There may be the loss or alteration of one or both breasts not to mention the loss of our hair. Just getting older is hard enough, but now we have to assimilate these changes all at once.

But gradually, our libido comes back, if we're patient and listen to our bodies. We will sense what we want from the sexual smorgasbord, whether it's cuddling or intercourse, and when.

I anticipate a more varied and tender sex life.

Avoidance

Avoidance is only a vacuum
that something else must fill.
Shirley Hazzard

While mastectomy had no impact on my undressing in front of my husband or on being nude in bed, my seeming physical openness is misleading. I have been undressing in front of my husband for twenty years, and that part is routine. But even though I'm nude, the actual act of making love is something else altogether. For now, we both practice avoidance. I don't like being caressed because it feels awkward, and I've told him so. Avoidance is how I've reconciled this feeling of being mutilated, despite the fact that I'm not physically covered up. Based on my experience, I would say that nudity does not equal adjustment.

༄

I am willing, but not yet able, to overcome my feeling that I've been disfigured.

Insecurity

What we suffer, what we endure . . . is done by us,
as individuals, in private.

Louise Bogan

At first I was willing to make love only as long as he couldn't see me. I always had a nightgown on—something, anything. It would slide, pull, move, but as long as I had a piece of clothing around me, I felt protected.

More often than not, covering up is our own form of psychic protection, a coping strategy that sometimes hardens into an unsatisfactory way of life when we find ourselves clinging to a cover-up like a suit of armor, months and even years later.

It is fair to say that failure to "show," like the failure to "tell," is a warning sign of an emotional impasse. Each of us must look at our own insecurities and ask in our heart of hearts if covering up has gone on too long.

✿

I will overcome my insecurities about my body
by facing them, not covering them up.

Performance Anxiety

Anxiety is love's greatest killer . . .

Anaïs Nin

We associate the term "performance anxiety" with a man's struggle to maintain an erect penis. But with doubts about our desirability and our deep-seated fears of rejection, is it possible that we, too, have developed a kind of performance anxiety?

Just as with men, the very risks we need to take to break the cycle of fear that paralyzes us are the risks we fear the most. Create safe boundaries and ease into them slowly. Perhaps stipulate that intercourse is not the aim. Try massage or gentle touching, and simply enjoy the pleasures of tactile sensations as a way to overcome the anxiety about how your body looks. Focus on the feelings.

Sensation keeps me in the present moment, far from anxiety about how I look.

Initiation

Freedom breeds freedom. Nothing else does.
Anne Roe

We make a good case for why our partners should make the first move. *I have been hurt by breast cancer, my self-image shattered,* we say to ourselves. *I need the reassurance of being truly wanted and desired. Without that, how can I feel desirable again?*

But inside our partner's mind and heart, there are also doubts and concerns: "She is in pain. She is sad. She will tell me when she is ready. I want to be sensitive and not impose myself on her."

We are the ones who have undergone this change. We know what we need and when. The way to get the reassurance we seek is to end the silence and assume the responsibility of opening up the dialogue.

～

I break the silence surrounding sexuality and speak of my own wants, fears, and needs.

Reactions

Perhaps it is the expediency in the . . .
eye that blinds it.

Virgilia Peterson

I had been nervously anticipating this moment in the bedroom. I thought I had a monopoly on doubt and insecurity. I didn't. My partner knew even less about what to do or what to say than I did. I never anticipated the complexity of his reactions, or that he might want me to help him deal with the changes to my body and our relationship brought on by my breast cancer.

There I was, looking for some assurance about my own worth and desirability, but I discovered he had needs of his own.

⁊

I am not the only one who needs reassurance about resuming our sex life.

Support for Men

Opening the window, I open myself.
Natalya Gorbanevskaya

My husband has been very affected by my cancer. He has realized that I may not be around, although I plan to be. Because of his sense of loss, his sexual desire has diminished and I am left to deal with the double whammy of needing more closeness *and* trying to understand his physical rejection.

I am not an island, but my husband wants to pretend he is. He hasn't acknowledged the changes in me or in our relationship, and if I start to talk about it he gets angry. We need more communication, but I can't do it alone. It is clear to me that men need to talk to each other and get support, just as women do. I have taken to putting brochures around the house that describe post-mastectomy counseling services, hoping he will seek the help he needs.

I can only open the window onto myself, opening up the possibility that others may pass through it, too.

Rejection

*The distance is nothing:
it is only the first step that is difficult.*

Marie Anne du Deffand

The first couple of months after my mastectomy, my husband said he was afraid of hurting me. I told him it was okay. Then he said that the worry prevented him from getting aroused. He started to come home late and fall asleep on the couch. We grew apart emotionally.

Later, he owned up that he was trying to get me to leave him so he could be done with the whole mess. He had married a pretty, perky, beauty queen and I was no longer that girl. But he felt he would be an outcast if he left me, and he'd have to live with the guilt. It took me one whole year of my life to realize that no matter what I felt like because of cancer and mastectomy, I didn't deserve sexual and emotional rejection. I finally gave him what he wanted. I walked out.

❧

Even painful experiences offer potential for change, growth, and a better life.

Reconciliation

*In some basic way it is our imperfection
and even our pain that draws others close to us.*
Rachel Naomi Remen

I was never obsessed about my looks and I didn't worry about my real and imagined flaws. Breast cancer took all that away. I remember looking in the mirror for the first time at my scarred, blank chest. I had decided that reconstruction wasn't for me. But now I didn't see a confident survivor. I saw ugliness and rejection. How could my partner accept this?

It took time for me to get used to my new body; how it felt to look at myself naked, to wash my chest, and how I looked in my clothes. But I found that as I grew more comfortable with my changed self, so did my partner who, soon, was no longer afraid to touch me and hold me close, grateful that I'm still here.

I accept and love myself as I am and trust that
others will accept and love me too.

Single Women

The age we call awkward
and the growing pains it inflicts . . .

Colette

As single women, we face great emotional risks following treatment for breast cancer. We are like teenagers again, self-conscious and insecure about what we have to offer to a partner. At the same time that our self-image has been threatened, we lay ourselves open to the challenges of dating. We question our desirability, but in this case we wonder, *Can anyone tell by looking at me that I've had a breast removed?* or, *Why would anyone want me once they find out I've had breast cancer?*

In seeking any new relationship, doubts about our attractiveness may surface.

And just like when we were teenagers, we feel a sense of joy and success when the person we desire responds with a gesture of interest and acceptance.

I trust that my insecurity will be overcome by my courage.

Hiding

The foolish vanity,
whence originates so many stratagems . . .

Charlotte Smith

My new boyfriend was in bed and I was in the bathroom brushing my teeth. When I finished, I took my clothes off and walked into the bedroom. My mind was a million miles away and I totally forgot that I was stark naked. I just strolled out, and he looked up at me in a very peculiar way. He had never seen me nude before. When I realized what I had done, I gasped, "Oh, no!" and tried to cover myself. He said, "What are you doing? Just come over here."

I went and stood by the bed for a moment and he looked at me, and the scar. He said, "That really looks okay. Please get in bed." And that was the end of it. From that moment on, the need to cover up my body was over and done.

Nothing is more healing than acceptance for who and what we are.

Risking New Relationships

What is life but one long risk?
Dorothy Canfield Fisher

Following breast cancer, a single woman may perceive everything as a risk. Every action in the direction of reaching out to others feels like a gamble. *If he doesn't want to see me again, how will I handle it? If I tell him, will he run?*

Instead, begin to view this process as a self-affirming one. We are taking care of our need to grow and change. We are proving our self-respect by being willing to risk. We are confident that if we are disappointed, we will not only survive, but we will try, try again.

I am getting on with my life unstopped by the judgments of others.

Withdrawal

I ain't had no loving since God knows when . . .
Gertrude "Ma" Rainey

The last thing on my mind when I was fighting breast cancer was sex. My sex life always seemed to be a feast or famine proposition, so the long dry spell through treatment and early recovery wasn't that tough. But as I was celebrating my first year anniversary of the end of chemo, I wondered if the long months with no sex were bad luck, or by choice. I thought about the last time I had sex. It was with the boyfriend who broke up with me right after my diagnosis. I remembered the anger. Now the pain hit me full force. I suddenly realized that I had reclaimed my health, but I had yet to reclaim my loving, sexual self.

I work on healing my whole being so that I may
feel desire, and desirable, once more.

Social Life

Now suddenly she was somebody, and as imprisoned in her difference as she had been in her anonymity.
Tillie Olsen

Fear of socializing may signal a fear of rejection. Beneath the layers of our conscious excuses we may believe that we are no longer attractive or desirable. We feel we are perpetuating a sham, passing for normal, when just below the surface is evidence that we are not.

Cloistering ourselves is one coping device. But by cutting ourselves off from social situations, we run the risk of undermining, not protecting, our fragile self-images.

Social situations are a testing ground and a way to regain confidence that despite our fears, we are not marked by a big C across our forehead or on our chest. Getting out and about is an important way to rebuild our self-esteem as we blend in, amuse, attract, and become the social, sexual self we once were.

I resist becoming a prisoner of my own fear by engaging socially.

Self-Esteem

The only one who can save me is me.

Karen Casey

We often project onto others what we believe about ourselves, including our self-criticisms. We expect to be rejected because we have rejected ourselves. Maybe we've given up because we are so demoralized that life dealt us the breast cancer hand. Why would someone want us now? What do we have to offer?

We learn to answer such real or implied questions positively as soon as we recognize that what we project into the world is what we see reflected back. Acceptance from others begins with acceptance of self. Love of others begins with love of self. New relationships begin, with or without breasts, with acceptance and love of self.

I must be there for myself before anyone can be there for me.

Self-Involvement

You need somebody to love you
while you're looking for someone to love.
Shelagh Delaney

For me, making love with a new partner was about testing my self-image, about putting an end to my identity crisis. I'm sure it's no different than it might be for a woman who seeks to begin a new relationship after divorce or widowhood. There is a transition phase after any life-altering event. It is initially less about loving someone else and more about finding ourselves again.

I acknowledge that sleeping with someone new
is, in part, a search for my own identity.

Resolution

*You need only claim the events of your life
to make yourself yours.*
Florida Scott-Maxwell

Sharing news of our breast cancer and the physical changes we have undergone is a moment of great courage and risk. It is standing up and saying, "This is who I am and it's okay," while facing the fear of possible rejection. In the moment that we tell in earnest, we learn something surprising: the reaction is actually inconsequential. When we are truly comfortable with ourselves, we experience only the rush of our personal power as we tell. True, it comes against the backdrop of all our struggles to get there. We may once have used verbal aggression to drive others away, or we were silent, not trusting that anyone could understand.

By deciding to take the risk to share, we experience the resolution that has gradually taken place inside us. A day comes when we are able to courageously tell our story and hear the response, knowing full well that whatever the reaction, we can handle it.

Today I tell and risk sharing a part of myself.

Second Chances

No person could save another.
                              Joyce Carol Oates

When we are diagnosed with breast cancer, we turn for help to those who can heal us. But even the most competent, sought-after doctors know that we are the ones who must do the hard work of surviving. We consider the options, choose our medicine, and will ourselves forward, in spite of our fears.

After treatment, the body slowly heals, but the emotional hurts, psychological confusion, and fear of recurrence may linger. Once again, we seek help, knowing it is up to us to do the hard work of healing. We consider our options, choose our path, and will ourselves forward, inspired by our second chance.

I ask for help, but it is up to me to heal my life.

Self-Awareness

Beginnings are apt to be shadowy.
Rachel Carson

Survivors come in many shapes, ages, attitudes, and personalities, and we have many different ideas about life after breast cancer. Some of us remain involved in support groups, others lead fundraising efforts, and many walk away, ready to put this experience in the past.

There is no one best way to transition to the next stage of our lives. We aren't required to wear the banner of "breast cancer survivor" across our chests. And we don't have to be a font of wisdom on life and death. The ordinary act of living a good and satisfying life is advice enough.

I live the life that is right for me, and I respect the choices other survivors make.

Checkups

What is out there is shaped by how we view it.
                                        Ellen J. Langer

We want black and white answers about the ongoing state of our disease, but doctors may give us answers shaded in grey, like "Current test results are of uncertain significance." That is a professional way of saying they can't be sure.

 What is certain is that we can choose our responses. After all, life is uncertain. What is significant is that we keep on living one day at a time, just like everyone else is doing.

I keep my eyes on what is in front of me, and enjoy this day.

Research

*For life today . . . is based on . . . ever-widening circles
of contact and communication.*

Anne Morrow Lindbergh

"Too much information" wasn't always a problem. In the past, it took hard work, persistence, and human connections to get answers about breast cancer. Fast forward to today. The Internet offers a world of "experts" instantly available at the touch of a finger. That's good news when sources are reliable and research-based. It's bad news when we find ourselves wandering from site to site, linking impulsively to questionable advice passing for truth, or scientific research we struggle to understand and apply.

As we move on in recovery, we use the tools at hand to monitor news about *surviving* breast cancer, but too much unfiltered information may bring both comfort and confusion. Our ongoing need for certainty underlies our constant searching. But soon we learn that the experts often have more questions than answers, just as we do.

I balance my need to know with my need to let go.

Recurrence

Just go for it. Life is a terminal condition.
Cancer patients just have more information.

Kris Carr

We grew up being told that you die of cancer. Today we know that you can live with cancer. That's what I am doing. Treatment—the handling and managing of my disease—will go on. But so will I. I'm not fighting anymore, but that doesn't mean I've given up. Far from it. I'm putting cancer in the background with all the other things that distract me from this moment. My eyes and my energy are focused on what I intend to do today.

I am living my life, moment to moment.

Loss of Friends

There are blessings and wonders
and horrific bad luck and no guarantees.
Barbara Kingsolver

Days and weeks go by when I don't think about cancer. I'm no longer obsessed with the odds of it coming back. I wake most mornings with a deeper sense of what a gift it is to make coffee or walk the dog. The hardest moments now are when I hear of the death of one of the wonderful women I've met through this experience. A kaleidoscope of emotions spins me around as her face comes into focus, and I hear her voice, her laugh.

I hold her there for a moment, remembering when I thought I couldn't take another step, how she carried me forward.

I cherish the gift of meeting my sister-travelers
and I endure the sorrow of their passing.

Insights

Pare your beliefs, your absolutes.
Make it simple . . . no carry-on luggage allowed.
Sheri Hostetler

We carry our habits and histories with us into this struggle, and we come out with more. After the dust has settled and we can see more clearly, we take a mental inventory of the people and things that got us through, and the ones that got in the way. The results can surprise us. What once were necessities can feel like burdens. A person we called friend or lover may now feel like a stranger. We didn't expect these changes, but we didn't expect breast cancer either.

There is a calm clarity that comes with an open, honest assessment of our experiences, and it readies us for the next step—to leave behind what no longer works and take with us what does.

What do I carry forward, and what do I set down?

Reflection

Heal your life and your life heals you.
Deena Metzger

Just as our eyes adjust to darkness and we begin to see the shape of things around us, we adjust to life after a breast cancer diagnosis. Slowly the view brightens, and we see that cancer will not be our undoing; our inability to move through its shadows will.

A sabbatical would be nice, but few of us can take all the time we'd like to reflect on what we've experienced and bring its impact into clearer focus. We can take a few, quiet moments each day or week to look at where we've been, where we are now, and where we want to go.

In looking back, I envision possibilities for going forward.

Part III.

A New Normal
A Time to Live

Reentry

*For a little while, this is the place for us——a place
of beginning things——and of ending things
I never thought would end.*

Beryl Markham

We want to "get back to normal" as soon as possible, but we
soon discover that we have fallen out of step with the familiar rhythms of family and work life. Things have changed
and we are renegotiating so much, from our responsibilities
to our relationships.

Reentry isn't always an easy path to travel. But with a
patience and creativity born of necessity, we adapt to cancer's impact on our lives. We let go of old routines and begin
to move forward, giving shape to our new normal.

I see more clearly what has ended in my life
because of cancer, and I begin again.

Uncertainty

It isn't for the moment you are stuck
that you need courage, but for the long uphill climb
back to sanity and faith and security.
Anne Morrow Lindbergh

The line dividing cancer *patient* from cancer *survivor* may be clearer to our doctors, family, and friends than it is to us. We're back on familiar ground but it may now feel like foreign ground. We wonder if we are seeing life clearly. We feel like we're losing our grip as we try to wake up from the nightmare of breast cancer, safe and sound.

The shock and disorientation a cancer diagnosis brings can fade into the background during grueling months of treatment. The reality of what we've been through may not sink in until we're home when, beyond the losses already tallied, we count another—a sense of certainty. Our bodies have been through so much, revealing how fragile and unpredictable life is. Our hearts and minds need time to catch up.

I trust I will feel at home in my life again.

Unraveling

You can make a perfect plan, and see it all unravel.
Lynn Miles

Wherever we are in life and whatever we're doing, we didn't plan on breast cancer. Our life unravels when we get this disease. The threads of our hopes and dreams unbraid and dangle like wisps of chemo-ravaged hair. We try to imagine how we're going to put it all back together.

Unraveling is an opportunity to see again—to *revision*—the beliefs, ideas, and goals woven so deeply within us that we've come to take them for granted. Unraveling is an opportunity to ask ourselves: *Will I keep all the colored threads of my past? What would the pattern reveal if I let go of the old and rewove a few, new threads into my life? What do I want my life to look like now?*

I reweave the fabric of my life in vital and cre-ative ways.

Next Steps

My life is, in fact, a continuous series of thresholds,
from one moment to the next . . .

Gunilla Norris

We're diagnosed, we walk straight into the thunderstorm of treatment, and we're awed by the lightning strikes a human body can withstand. We wonder who will be the last one standing, breast cancer or us. We're suspended between what was and what comes next. We wait it out, this abundance of loss. Time passes, and our appetite for life returns. We get up and cross over once again, to our present.

I step into now.

Moving On

. . . we are voyagers, discoverers of the not-known,
the unrecorded; we have no map . . .

H.D.

There are no guidebooks describing exactly where to go from here, how to get there, or what we'll find when we do. We are standing on a shoreline, a mesmerizing place where land and ocean meet. Is this the place where land ends and ocean begins, or is it the other way around?

Life itself moves like the meeting of waves and shore, a perpetual rhythm of endings and beginnings. Through the peaceful sojourns, troubling detours, and unexpected stops, we map each step along the way, writing the guides to our unique journeys.

I welcome each departure, arrival, and all the space in between.

Detachment

Peace, she supposed, was contingent upon a certain
disposition of the soul, a disposition to receive the gift
that only detachment from self made possible.

Elizabeth Goudge

Detachment from the pressure of whether or not we are doing "well enough" in life is one of the benefits a brush with cancer provides. We separate ourselves from our need to strive. We carefully consider where our energies go. This is neither "checking out" nor selfishness, but separation from the false urgencies of life. The insights that come from detachment provide me with a new standard by which to live.

I am more aware of what is truly meaningful to me.

Attention

There are no sick people in North Oxford.
They are either dead or alive.
It's sometimes difficult to tell the difference, that's all.
Barbara Pym

Now that we can tell the difference between what is dead and what is alive in our own lives, how can we afford to let fear dominate our days? Isn't there something else, something more precious to focus on? Take in all the bittersweet beauty of being alive. Pay attention to the small things, how the warmth of the sun feels on your skin, and how your shadow falls across the sidewalk. Take pleasure in the smile from a passing stranger. Yes, the clichés are true: in facing death, we have an opportunity to savor life.

I rediscover the beauty in what is in front of me this day.

Challenges

We could never learn to be brave and patient,
if there were only joy in the world.

Helen Keller

Breast cancer is nothing if not a training ground for learning to overcome fears, barriers, obstacles, and insecurities, one after another, learning to find our way over, under, or around them. Some obstacles simply evaporate in the face of cancer. Others, we master because of the urgency that cancer brings into our life. It's not that the fear goes away. But by now we are actually skilled at knowing how to overcome feelings of fear and helplessness. We are like medieval warriors with lance tilted, ever ready should new challenges present themselves.

In meeting the challenge of cancer, I strengthen my sense of self.

Humor

*Everyone's survival kit
should contain a sense of humor.*

Anonymous

There is a popular t-shirt among breast cancer survivors that says, "Yes, they're fake. The real ones tried to kill me." The first time I saw it I laughed without even thinking about it. That shirt said it all. I admired the courage and the attitude of the woman wearing it, and I thanked her for making my day.

Breast cancer takes so much from us, but if we can hang on to a sense of humor, it is easier to hang on to our hopes, plans, dreams, and joys in living each day.

Laughter heals and helps me to see the possibilities in life.

Self-Direction

I'll walk where my own nature would be leading;
it vexes me to choose another guide.

Emily Brontë

In times of tranquility, experience guides us. In times of suffering, experience propels us.

It's not that things are so different, but we see them in a different light, unfiltered by routine responsibilities and the compromises we make to get through each day.

We have made the hard choices, ones only we could make on behalf of our survival. We have come to know our fears and desires, inside and out. And we have been returned to ourselves, ready to choose what's right for us now.

I will lead my life in a direction of my own choosing.

Limitations

That is what learning is.
You suddenly understand something you've
understood all your life, but in a new way.

Doris Lessing

It was important to me that I approach the months of treatment almost in denial. It became mind over matter: go forward. My parents always told me I could do anything, and I succeeded at whatever I put my mind to. Why should cancer be any different? I had no time to dwell on *me*, only on what needed to be done.

I can tell you that I learned I have limitations I did not think existed. I learned that breast cancer wasn't a test I could pass or fail. It wasn't a race I could win or lose. It *was* a lesson in acceptance—I don't have all the answers, there are times when I need help, and it is okay to take care of *me*. That's how I'm approaching my life now.

I am proud of my strengths and I accept my limitations; both are part of me.

Perspective

I did not really like shipboard life
but the sea was a mighty experience.
                                    Florida Scott-Maxwell

My body, mind, and spirit have been sorely tested. I don't know what it all means. I don't know why I got breast cancer. I don't know why bad things happen to good people and good things happen to bad people. I do know that to be pulled out of eternity to voyage a while here is worth all the sickness we endure while we live.

✍

Oh, what an amazing journey I'm on!

Turning Point

Most turning points are evident only afterward.
Amanda Cross

I was ready to let go of the label, "survivor." It felt like a weight I didn't need to carry any longer. One day I left it behind, releasing the name that gave me an identity when I'd lost track of who I was before breast cancer.

As we go with the flow of life after cancer, it's hard to pinpoint the moment when we put it behind us. It's hard to say when life feels normal again. But that moment does come, like running into an old friend after a long absence and picking up where we left off, sharing old memories and making new ones.

I keep memories in their place, and welcome the chance to make new ones.

Arrival

Don't be afraid that your life will end;
be afraid that it will never begin.

Grace Hansen

There are women all around us who have experienced breast cancer. They are well acquainted with the temporary moorings that come with life—family, friends, home, work, marriage, children, health—until they're abruptly cut loose from familiar shores. They, too, lived through the season of fear, hanging on to plans and dreams. They, too, lived beyond the loss, letting go of things they no longer needed to carry, to arrive at new beginnings. We might notice them there—a glimmer of courage in an uncertain world.

I welcome my new beginning, knowing I am in good company.

Self-Discovery

. . . there is only movement through the labyrinth
of experience until we remember who we really are.
Twyla Hurd Nitsch, Seneca Elder

It has been thirty-five years since my beginning steps on this road. I am not the person I was before breast cancer. I am physically, emotionally, mentally, and spiritually stronger.

I look back and wonder at my self-centeredness. Cancer took me on a journey from being concerned about how I looked, what I had, and who I was hanging out with, to what I think of as the real life issues for me: my family, my friends, my health, and my spirituality.

Something, and I call it God, gave me the impression that I would be okay. But I still had to walk through the labyrinth of life and death issues. I might have matured as well in a normal, non-threatening world, but surviving cancer made me like myself more. I stopped wasting time on how I looked and discovered who I was, and who I might become.

I am still here and getting to know myself better each day.

Living with Metastatic Cancer

Don't put off your happy life.

Anonymous

It would be nice if, like in childhood fairy tales, a knight would ride in to slay the dragon of metastatic breast cancer. But I know cancer is here to stay. It terrifies me to make peace with this beast and once again, defend myself with all the bravery I can muster. But I do, for in this world, no one lives "happily ever after." Each of our stories will end. But I will live happily, even knowing that cancer will be a bigger part of my tale than I had ever imagined.

I face the facts, feel the fear, and go on living.

Time

One day . . . one whole day with its night passes.
It is a whole lifetime.

Gunilla Norris

As we grow older, time seems to move faster. Life picks up speed as we rush closer to the end of our earthly days. But no matter how old we are, breast cancer can make us feel the same way: *It's all happening so fast. Where did the time go? How much more do I get?*

We all want more time, of course, even though we spend much of it distracted by what has already happened, or what we wish would happen. Cancer reminds us that life is lived in the present tense. And just as a life can be long in years but short on living, so may a life be short in years, but long in its living.

I live this day.

Opportunity

There are more awakenings than births in a life.
Carolyn Heilbrun

How does a major illness become an advantage? It starts with a keen appreciation of life. It deepens into a release—a letting go, not of life, but of all the petty annoyances that once clouded our view of the transitory nature of things. As the importance of things recedes, the importance of relationships comes to the fore. We set about them with a heightened intensity. We *really* have them. We know what we feel and we say what we think. We know what it is we wish to accomplish. There are equal amounts of pain and joy in every moment, and ironically, we feel ourselves more awake and alive than ever before. We have found a new way of being in the present.

I embrace the opportunity to find out who I really am.

Transformation

*The old woman I shall become will be quite different
from the woman I am now. Another I is beginning.*
                                        George Sand

We have lived beyond breast cancer. It is part of our story, but it's not the whole story. We've survived many things in life. Some experiences challenged us. Others transformed us.

For many of us, breast cancer is transformative. We learn to pull all the parts of ourselves—body, mind, and spirit—together as this disease teaches us to hold on and to let go, to laugh and to cry, to question and to believe. It teaches us to fight and to make peace with what is. Most of all, it teaches us to live each moment while looking in the face of death.

I embrace the transformative lessons that breast
cancer offers.

Alive

I used to trouble what life was for—now
being alive seems sufficient reason.

Joanna Field

"What's happening in your life?"

"I'm alive!"

⁂

I am alive this moment and it is enough.

About the Authors

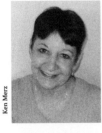

Ken Merz

Pat Benson provides freelance writing and editing services to clients whose work promotes personal growth and a more compassionate world. She is the former Rights Director at Hazelden Publishing in Minnesota, whose products help people understand and overcome addiction and encourage personal and spiritual development. This is her first book.

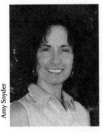

Amy Snyder

Linda Dackman is the author of *Up Front: Sex and the Post-Mastectomy Woman* and *Affirmations, Meditations, and Encouragements for Women Living with Breast Cancer.* She has been a peer counselor for the American Cancer Society and is the Public information Director Emeritus for the Exploratorium, a museum of science and art in San Francisco. This is her third book.

To Our Readers

Conari Press, an imprint of Red Wheel/Weiser, publishes books on topics ranging from spirituality, personal growth, and relationships to women's issues, parenting, and social issues. Our mission is to publish quality books that will make a difference in people's lives—how we feel about ourselves and how we relate to one another. We value integrity, compassion, and receptivity, both in the books we publish and in the way we do business.

Our readers are our most important resource, and we appreciate your input, suggestions, and ideas about what you would like to see published.

Visit our website at *www.redwheelweiser.com* to learn about our upcoming books and free downloads, and be sure to go to *www.redwheelweiser.com/newsletter* to sign up for newsletters and exclusive offers.

You can also contact us at *info@rwwbooks.com*.

Conari Press
an imprint of Red Wheel/Weiser, LLC
665 Third Street, Suite 400
San Francisco, CA 94107